ASTAXANTHIN

A Comprehensive Guide To
Harnessing Nature's Most Potent
Antioxidant For Optimal Health,
Anti-Aging, And Peak Performance

SAMANTHA ZYLAR

Contents

CHAPTER ONE

Overview

There are certain hidden gems in the realm of natural compounds that have many amazing qualities, even if they are concealed from view. A bright red carotenoid pigment called astaxanthin is one such undiscovered nutritional and health benefit. Astaxanthin, which is derived from a variety of plants, microbes, and marine life, is becoming more and more well-known for its powerful antioxidant qualities and many health advantages.

The genius of astaxanthin is its capacity to impart red and pink tones to all aspects of the natural world, including the flesh of salmon and the plumage of flamingos. Many aquatic organisms have beautiful colors and can resist harsh climatic conditions because of this chemical. Researchers, health enthusiasts, and consumers have all taken notice of it as they realize how beneficial it could be for improving human health and well-being.

Astaxanthin is a member of the carotenoids family, which is a pigment family renowned for its anti-oxidant qualities. But astaxanthin is unique because of how powerful it is. It is frequently regarded as one of nature's most powerful antioxidants.

Its potential to shield cells, tissues, and essential organs from the damaging effects of aging and chronic diseases has garnered attention due to its capacity to counteract oxidative stress and inflammation.

Astaxanthin is a hidden gem that is beginning to get the recognition it deserves in the domains of exercise research, cosmetics, and nutrition. Nowadays, this carotenoid can be easily accessed by people through a variety of forms, such as topical treatments and supplements. Astaxanthin is becoming more and more popular because of its intense antioxidant properties as well as its ability to promote eye health, improve the complexion of the skin, increase athletic performance, and even lower the risk of chronic diseases.

The sources, health advantages, and possible uses of astaxanthin will all be covered in this article. It will illuminate this hidden jewel of nature's various facets, from its function in the natural world to its growing importance for human health and wellbeing. Whether you are a scientist looking for new ways to decipher the secrets of this bright molecule or a health-conscious consumer, astaxanthin looks to be a fascinating topic of study and a promising addition to your nutritional program.

Founding Of Astaxanthin:

Many different types of creatures contain astaxanthin, a deep reddish-orange carotenoid pigment that occurs naturally. The following can be used to summarize its exploration and discovery:

1. What Is The Word Astaxanthin:

The word "astaxanthin," which is pronounced "asta-zan-thin," comes from the Haematococcus species of microalgae, which is one of the main naturally-occurring producers of this pigment. Specifically, the microalga Haematococcus pluvialis is able to collect astaxanthin in response to a variety of stresses, including intense light or nutritional shortage. It is thought that this adaptation shields the algae from UV light and oxidative damage.

2. Early Investigation And Study:

• Microalga Discovery: Haematococcus pluvialis was identified as the source of astaxanthin, owing to its distinct capacity to yield this vivid pigment. The alga's ability to adapt to stressful environments prompted research into it as a possible astaxanthin source.

• Salmon Pigmentation: Scientists noticed that after ingesting Haematococcus pluvialis or other astaxanthin-containing species, salmon and other aquatic creatures, such as shrimp and flamingos, gained their characteristic pink or red hue. This phenomenon aroused scientific interest, leading to investigations into the pigment's origin.

• Synthetic synthesis: As scientific understanding grew, astaxanthin synthesis techniques were created. This made it possible to create astaxanthin supplements, which are currently widely utilized in the aquaculture sector to improve the color of fish and crustaceans that are raised. Additionally, because of its possible antioxidant qualities and other health advantages, astaxanthin pills have become more and more well-liked in the health and wellness industry.

• Applications: Astaxanthin, which is used in aquaculture and dietary supplements, is also used in skincare and cosmetics. Its antioxidant qualities are thought to provide anti-aging and protective effects for the skin.

In conclusion, astaxanthin was first discovered by its observation in microalgae such as Haematococcus pluvialis, and its function in the vivid coloring of several aquatic animals. Research and development over time resulted in the synthesis of astaxanthin and its use in a range of sectors, including cosmetics and aquaculture.

The Mechanisms Of Astaxanthin Science

Known for its vivid red color, astaxanthin is a naturally occurring carotenoid with strong antioxidant qualities. It is present in a variety of marine creatures and has drawn interest recently because of its health advantages. Examining astaxanthin's composition and sources is crucial to comprehending the science underlying it.

Comprehending Astaxanthin's Chemistry:

1. Chemical Structure: Because of its chemical makeup, astaxanthin is distinct among carotenoid pigments. It is made up of 40 carbon atoms twisted into a lengthy chain with many functional groups that hold oxygen. Its exceptional antioxidant activity

can be attributed to this complicated structure.

2. Properties of an Antioxidant: Resistant to free radicals and reactive oxygen species (ROS), astaxanthin is a potent antioxidant. Because of its capacity to neutralize these dangerous substances, it may be able to shield tissues and cells against oxidative damage, a condition linked to a number of health problems, including aging and chronic illnesses.

3. Quenching Singlet Oxygen: Research has demonstrated that astaxanthin is especially efficient at squelching singlet oxygen, a highly reactive type of oxygen that can lead

to oxidative stress. Because of its capacity to neutralize singlet oxygen, astaxanthin is regarded as a superior antioxidant.

4. Astaxanthin provides cellular protection by accumulating in mitochondria and cell membranes, where it prevents oxidative damage to these essential biological components. Astaxanthin can cross cell membranes. Because of this, it is an important part of maintaining overall cellular health.

Where To Find Astaxanthin?

1. Microalgae: Haematococcus pluvialis and other microalgae are the

principal producers of astaxanthin. As a defense against hostile environmental factors including high sunshine and nutrient deprivation, these microalgae build up astaxanthin.

2. Astaxanthin-rich microalgae are the food source for krill, a type of microscopic crustacean that builds up this substance inside of their bodies. Astaxanthin can be found in krill oil, which is frequently included in nutritional supplements.

3. Salmon and Trout: Astaxanthin is predominantly obtained by wild salmon and trout through their diet, which includes krill and other astaxanthin-rich marine creatures.

This explains the unique pinkish-red coloring of these fish.

4. Synthetic Production: Although natural sources are normally favored due to their bioavailability and potential for higher quality goods, astaxanthin can also be synthesized synthetically utilizing petrochemicals.

In conclusion, astaxanthin's distinct molecular structure and exceptional antioxidant qualities are the main foci of its scientific research. It has numerous possible health advantages, such as promoting skin and eye health and lowering the risk of chronic illnesses.

To fully utilize its potential in dietary supplements, cosmetics, and aquaculture, among other applications, it is imperative to comprehend its chemistry and sources.

CHAPTER TWO

Benefits Of Astaxanthin For Health

1. Antioxidant: One of nature's most powerful antioxidants is astaxanthin, a powerful antioxidant. It aids in defending tissues and cells from oxidative damage brought on by free radicals. This can improve general health and lower the chance of developing chronic illnesses.

2. Effects On Inflammation: Astaxanthin has shown strong anti-inflammatory qualities. It may be able to lessen the symptoms of inflammatory illnesses like arthritis by lowering inflammation levels in the body.

3. Skin And Eye Health:

Astaxanthin has a reputation for improving both the condition of the skin and the eyes. It can lessen the visibility of wrinkles and increase the suppleness and moisture content of the skin. Furthermore, it could promote eye health by shielding the eyes from UV rays and oxidative stress, which could lower the chance of developing age-related eye disorders.

4. Benefits For The Cardiovascular System:

Astaxanthin can protect the cardiovascular system by lowering oxidative stress, a significant cause of heart disease. It has been linked to better blood vessel function, lowered blood pressure, and improved lipid profiles—all of which can promote heart health.

To get these health benefits, you can consider including astaxanthin in your diet or taking it as a dietary supplement. Before incorporating any new supplement into your regimen, you should always speak with a healthcare provider, especially if you have any underlying medical concerns or are on medication.

Nutrition And Astaxanthin

The potential health advantages of astaxanthin, a powerful antioxidant, and carotenoid, have made it more well-known in recent years. It is a naturally occurring substance that is present in many aquatic species, particularly microalgae and is essential to both aquatic life and human nutrition. We'll look at its dietary sources, suggested daily consumption, and supplementation here.

Food-Based Sources

1. Microalgae: When subjected to environmental stressors like UV radiation, microalgae like Haematococcus pluvialis create huge amounts of astaxanthin, which is the primary source of astaxanthin. Because astaxanthin is accumulated by fish and crustaceans through their consumption of these algae, seafood has higher quantities of it.

2. Seafood: The most well-known dietary sources of astaxanthin include lobster, shrimp, trout, and salmon. Particularly wild-caught salmon is prized for having a high astaxanthin

concentration, which gives it a pink or reddish hue.

3. Another source of astaxanthin is krill oil, which is derived from the microscopic crustaceans known as krill that resemble shrimp. Because of its high astaxanthin and omega-3 fatty acid content, this oil is utilized as a nutritional supplement.

Suggested Daily Consumption:

Consumption: The suggested daily consumption of astaxanthin is contingent upon personal characteristics, including age, gender, and health objectives. As with certain vitamins and minerals, astaxanthin does not have an official Recommended Dietary Allowance (RDA). However, according to scientists, eating a range of foods high in astaxanthin can be good for your general health. Here are a few broad recommendations:

1. Dietary Consumption: There are advantages to regularly including foods high in astaxanthin in your diet. A few times a week of eating seafood, such as wild-caught salmon, can help maintain healthy astaxanthin consumption.

2. Supplements and Dosage: For people who might not obtain enough

astaxanthin from their food or who want to focus on certain health issues, supplements are offered. Dosages may vary depending on the product and the intended function.

The typical range of supplement dosages is 4 to 12 milligrams per day; however, since every person's needs are different, it is imperative to speak with a healthcare provider before beginning any new supplement regimen.

While astaxanthin is generally thought to be safe when taken as directed, high quantities have the potential to cause negative effects or conflict with specific drugs. Before taking astaxanthin supplements, people who are breastfeeding or pregnant, as well as those with certain medical conditions, should consult a doctor.

In conclusion, astaxanthin's potent antioxidant qualities make it an important part of the diet. Supplements are available, however, dietary sources such as seafood and krill oil can also provide it. Including astaxanthin in your diet in a balanced and knowledgeable way may provide a number of health benefits, but you should be aware of the right dosages and speak with a doctor if you have any questions about its use.

CHAPTER THREE

Skincare & Beauty With Astaxanthin

1. A Natural Remedy For Youthful Skin:

Rich in carotenoid and antioxidant properties, astaxanthin has several advantages for skincare and cosmetics. By scavenging free radicals that can harm skin and hasten the appearance of wrinkles, it aids in the fight against aging. A more youthful complexion can be achieved through topical treatments or regular usage of astaxanthin tablets.

2. The Function Of Astaxanthin In Sunscreen:

Due to its capacity to offer organic sun protection, Astaxanthin has drawn notice. Although astaxanthin cannot completely replace conventional sunscreen, it can strengthen the skin's barrier against UV rays and reduce the harm they can do. It is a useful supplement to a sun protection routine since it lowers the risk of skin cancer, sunburn, and skin redness.

3. Cosmetics & Beauty Goods:

Astaxanthin is being used

in more and more cosmetics and beauty goods. It is present in creams, serums, and other skincare products. Its antioxidant qualities aid in reducing hyperpigmentation, enhancing moisture retention, and improving the texture of the skin. Because astaxanthin reduces inflammation, it is beneficial for relieving sensitive or irritated skin. It is frequently promoted as an active component of moisturizing, regenerating, and anti-aging cosmetics.

In conclusion, astaxanthin has a variety of applications in skincare and cosmetics. In order to help people obtain healthier, and more young, and beautiful skin, it provides natural anti-aging qualities, helps protect skin from the sun, and is used in a variety of cosmetic products.

Astaxanthin In Exercise And Sports

A natural pigment and strong antioxidant present in many marine creatures, astaxanthin has drawn a lot of interest recently due to its possible advantages in the field of sports and fitness. This carotenoid is highly recognized for its ability to improve muscle health and performance, increase endurance and recuperation, and even draw attention from athletes as a supplement with scientific backing. Let's explore each of these facets individually:

1. Boosting Endurance And Recovery:

Astaxanthin's remarkable antioxidant qualities are well-known, and they can aid in lowering the body's level of oxidative stress. This is especially helpful for athletes who play endurance sports like swimming, cycling, or long-distance running. Extended physical activity can produce inflammation and free radicals, which can wear down muscles and slow down the healing process. Because astaxanthin can neutralize these dangerous chemicals, it can help maintain endurance by speeding up the recovery process after a workout and minimizing muscle damage.

2. Muscle Function And Health: Astaxanthin may be very important for maintaining the health and function of muscles. It's a tempting choice for people who want to get the most out of their exercises or sports because it may improve muscle strength and endurance. This carotenoid aids in reducing inflammation and discomfort in the muscles, hastening recuperation and maybe enhancing general muscle performance.

3. The Science Of Athlete Endorsements:

Numerous well-known athletes have expressed interest in astaxanthin as additional research on its possible health benefits for athletes is being done. The sports and fitness community has seen a rise in the use of astaxanthin supplements as a result of these endorsements. Athlete recommendations also draw attention to how crucial it is to use supplements with scientific backing to enhance performance and recuperation.

Although astaxanthin's benefits for sports and fitness are supported by promising scientific research, it's crucial to remember that individual reactions may differ. To find the best dosages and usage schedules, athletes and fitness enthusiasts should speak with medical professionals or sports nutritionists. Furthermore, rather than being the only supplement used to boost performance, astaxanthin should be seen as an additional element of a healthy diet and exercise regimen.

In conclusion, astaxanthin is a fascinating supplement for anyone interested in sports and fitness because of its capacity to boost endurance, quicken recovery, and increase muscle health and performance. Astaxanthin's growing renown, supported by data from studies and athlete recommendations, indicates that it might be a useful supplement for enhancing sports performance as well as general health and wellness. Like any supplement, though, it should only be taken sparingly and after consulting a healthcare provider.

Aquaculture And Agriculture Using Astaxanthin

Because of its many advantages, astaxanthin is a naturally occurring carotenoid pigment that is important to both aquaculture and agriculture.

1. Fish Farming And Aquaculture Using Astaxanthin:

• Color Enhancement: In fish farming, astaxanthin is frequently used to improve the color of fish, especially salmon and trout. Customers will find the fish more enticing since it gives the flesh a vivid pink or crimson color.

• Antioxidant Properties: Astaxanthin is a potent antioxidant that helps guard farmed fish against illness and oxidative stress. The fish's immune system is strengthened, increasing their resistance to illness.

• Growth and Reproduction: In certain species, astaxanthin can enhance growth rates and reproduction, which is essential for aquaculture operations to remain profitable.

• Nutritional Value: By improving the nutritional profile of fish, it helps consumers choose better options. Moreover, astaxanthin can take the place of artificial additives in fish feed, supporting the movement toward more sustainable and organic aquaculture methods.

2. Agriculture With Astaxanthin:

• It can assist in shielding crops from oxidative damage brought on by environmental stresses like UV radiation and extremely high or low temperatures when administered as a foliar spray or mixed into soil amendments.

• Yield Enhancement: Astaxanthin can increase crop yields by lowering plant stress. Additionally, it may enhance the quality of fruits and vegetables, raising their possible market worth.

• Disease Resistance: Astaxanthin can strengthen plants' immune systems, increasing their resistance to pests and illnesses, much like it does in aquaculture.

• Sustainable Agriculture: The natural sources of astaxanthin correspond with the increasing need for organic and sustainable farming methods. It provides a sustainable substitute for the artificial chemicals utilized in traditional farming.

The application of astaxanthin in aquaculture and agriculture shows how natural substances can enhance the well-being, aesthetics, and productivity of living things, whether they be fish or crops, while also supporting more ecologically friendly and sustainable methods.

CHAPTER FOUR

Astaxanthin In The Preservation Of The Environment

Naturally occurring carotenoid astaxanthin has gained attention for both its potential health benefits and environmental conservation value. Its effect on controlling algal blooms and its function in safeguarding ecosystems and wildlife are two crucial factors to take into account in this context.

1. Algal Blooms And Ecosystems:

Algal blooms pose a serious threat to the

environment because they are typified by the fast and uncontrollably growing algae in aquatic environments. Numerous negative consequences on ecosystems, such as habitat disruption, oxygen depletion, and the generation of toxic algal blooms, can result from these blooms.

Certain microalgae and krill produce astaxanthin, which has been connected to reducing the effects of algal blooms in a number of ways.

• Anti-Oxidative Properties: Microalgae's cell membranes store astaxanthin, a potent antioxidant that shields the organisms from oxidative stress. Maintaining control over these microalgae populations aids in preventing overdevelopment and the start of algal blooms.

• Decrease in Dangerous Algal Toxins: Astaxanthin may have a role in lowering the dangerous algal toxins generated during blooms.

It can neutralize reactive oxygen species, which frequently aid in the production of toxins because it is a strong antioxidant. It contributes to the preservation of aquatic ecosystem health by lowering toxic levels.

• Maintaining the Balance of the Food Chain: Astaxanthin-rich microalgae are a vital link in the aquatic food chain, giving zooplankton and other creatures a steady supply of food. Preserving this equilibrium is essential for the ecosystem's general well-being, as it averts disturbances brought about by the excessive numbers of specific species.

2. The Function Of Astaxanthin In Preserving Wildlife:

Preserving wildlife is essential to environmental health, and astaxanthin has demonstrated potential in this area as well. Astaxanthin is beneficial to a number of wildlife species, especially those that live in watery environments:

• Salmon and Trout: These fish species' vivid pink and red coloring is caused by astaxanthin. Their availability of foods high in astaxanthin in the wild supports biodiversity and helps keep populations stable.

• Crustaceans: The diets of crustaceans, such as shrimp, crabs, and lobsters, provide astaxanthin as well. It is this component that gives them their unique colors and general well-being. Wildlife that depends on these environments for survival is also indirectly protected when the ecosystems that support these species are preserved.

• Migrating birds: Occasionally, aquatic settings rich in astaxanthin might draw migrating birds by providing them with a plentiful food source. We can guarantee these birds' welfare throughout their yearly migrations by protecting these environments.

In conclusion, there is a great chance that astaxanthin will aid in environmental preservation. Its significance in preserving the delicate balance of ecosystems is highlighted by its function in averting and reducing algal blooms as well as by its beneficial effects on the well-being and sustainability of numerous wildlife species. The more we learn about astaxanthin's advantages, the more obvious it is that this organic substance can help preserve our ecosystem for coming generations.

A Prospect For Sustainability

Sustainability Practices:

Astaxanthin, a potent antioxidant and pigment present in certain seafood and microalgae, is garnering interest due to its potential to support sustainable development. Several astaxanthin-related sustainability measures consist of:

1. Aquaculture: To improve the color of farmed fish like salmon and trout, astaxanthin is frequently utilized in this field. In order to minimize their negative effects on the environment, sustainable aquaculture practices seek to reduce the usage of synthetic astaxanthin by investigating natural sources and optimizing feed formulas.

2. Natural Sources: To lessen the dependency on chemical manufacture, research is being done to find and utilize astaxanthin's natural sources, such as Haematococcus pluvialis microalgae. Because they lessen reliance on non-renewable resources and the carbon impact, these initiatives support sustainability goals.

3. The sustainable development of microalgae that are high in astaxanthin necessitates the use of closed-loop systems, resource optimization, and waste minimization. Efficient growth and extraction techniques are being developed to reduce water and energy use.

Future Research And Advancements:

The sustainable future of astaxanthin depends on continued research and advancements. Key areas of concentration include:

1. Improved Production Methods: Research intends to boost astaxanthin

production using biotechnology, genetic engineering, and selective breeding of microalgae. These technologies can boost yield while lowering resource inputs.

2. Waste Utilization: Finding novel ways to utilize byproducts of astaxanthin production, such as residual biomass, can limit waste and encourage circular economy practices.

3. Regulatory Frameworks: Developing clear standards and sustainability certifications for astaxanthin products can drive the industry toward more responsible practices and help customers make educated decisions.

4. Bioavailability Studies: Research on the bioavailability and health advantages of astaxanthin is crucial for promoting its use and encouraging its integration into nutraceuticals, eliminating the demand for synthetic colorants in numerous industries.

In conclusion, astaxanthin presents significant prospects for a sustainable future, notably in the aquaculture and nutraceutical sectors. By implementing more eco-friendly production methods and continuing research into its benefits and applications, we can lower the environmental footprint associated with this precious molecule and create a more sustainable future.

Conclusion

Astaxanthin is a carotenoid pigment and strong antioxidant that has become important in the field of nutrition and health. In retrospect, it is evident that the discovery of astaxanthin's extraordinary health advantages has sparked a revolution in the fields of natural medicine and dietary supplements.

Because of its exceptional capacity to fend against oxidative stress, lessen inflammation, and promote a host of human health benefits, astaxanthin is a highly sought-after substance. It has been demonstrated to increase cardiovascular health, strengthen skin health, improve eye function, and even speed up the healing process after physical activity. Its potential goes well beyond customary applications, as continued study uncovers new advantages and uses.

We look forward to seeing even more innovative advancements in astaxanthin usage and research in the future. Innovation and research are still motivated by the possibility of using this effective antioxidant in the management and prevention of a wide range of medical disorders. Astaxanthin is probably going to be very important for health and wellness in the future, from cosmetics to sports nutrition.

There is no indication that the Astaxanthin Revolution is slowing down, and exploring its potential will be just as fascinating as learning about the past. With astaxanthin's potential to improve our lives in a multitude of ways, we must continue to be aware of research findings and practice careful use as we go forward.

www.ingramcontent.com/pod-product-compliance
Lightning Source LLC
Chambersburg PA
CBHW060842260726

48661CB00002B/554